I0428806

The Ketogenic Diet for Beginners

The Basics of Ketosis and a Collection of Recipes

Table of Contents

Introduction 3

Chapter One: What is Ketosis? 4

    Benefits of Ketosis.. 4

Chapter Two: The Ketogenic Diet 6

    Creating a Ketogenic Diet 7

Chapter Three: Ketogenic Recipes 10

    Spiced Pumpkin Waffles 11

    Herbed Mushroom Omelet.. 13

    Almond Flour Blueberry Muffins 15

    Garlic Cheddar Biscuits 17

    Walnut, Apple Chicken Salad 19

    Creamy Avocado Soup 20

    Avocado Egg Salad 21

    Curried Lentil Soup.. 22

    Herb-Roasted Chicken Legs.. 24

    Balsamic Grilled Salmon Steaks 26

    Cheese-Stuffed Meatloaf 27

    Bacon-Wrapped Scallops 29

Conclusion... 30

Introduction

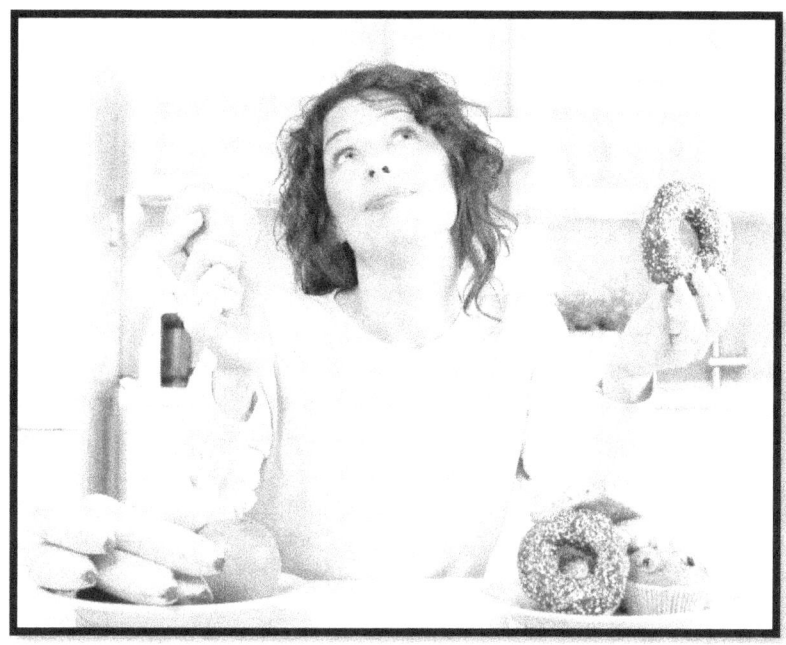

If you know anything about the ketogenic diet, you have probably heard that it is a type of low-carbohydrate diet. In reality, however, it is much more than that – it is a type of diet designed to encourage your body to burn stored fats for fuel, thus helping to improve your overall health and, potentially, speed your weight loss. The ketogenic diet has also been linked to relief from or reversal of symptoms for a number of serious health conditions including Type 2 diabetes, epilepsy and even cancer. If you are curious about what the ketogenic diet is and what it can do for you, this book is the perfect place to start. Within the pages of this book you will find information about the basics of the diet including how it works and its benefits. You will also find lists of foods to avoid and those you should eat when following a ketogenic diet. Finally, you will receive a collection of delicious recipes to help you get started on the ketogenic diet.

So what are you waiting for? Keep reading and get started on the ketogenic diet today!

Chapter One: What is Ketosis?

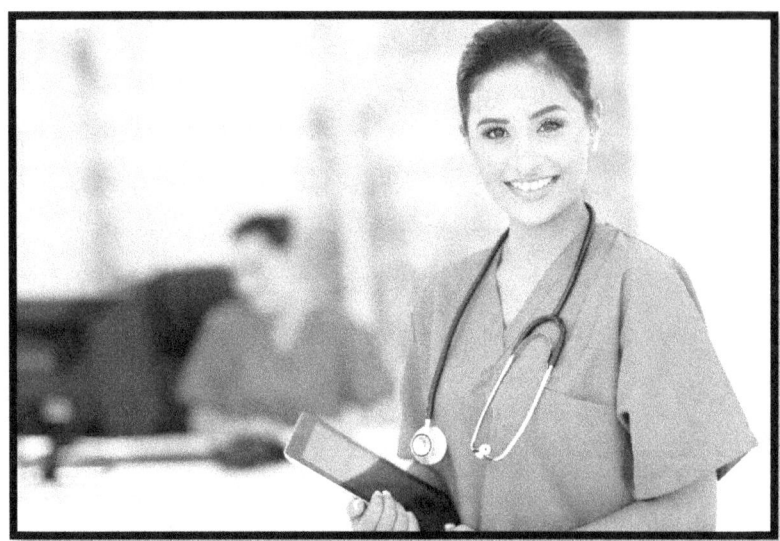

The term "ketosis" is associated with elevated levels of ketone bodies in the body and in the blood. Ketone bodies are formed when the glycogen stores in your liver are depleted – the ketone bodies are then used for energy. A state of ketosis in the body can be reached through fasting or by depriving the body of high-carbohydrate foods. When glucose is not regularly being consumed, typically in the form of high-carbohydrate foods, the body must start burning fat stores (ketone bodies) for fuel as an alternative. Eating more fats and protein than carbohydrates is the simplest way to encourage the body to enter a state of ketosis.

Benefits of Ketosis

There are a wide variety of benefits associated with a state of ketosis in the body – these benefits can apply to anyone, not just for diabetics who must follow a ketogenic diet for medical reasons. Some of the benefits of ketosis for the body include:

- Relief from or reversal of Type 2 diabetes symptoms
- Improves treatment for epilepsy patients, may help reduce frequency/severity of seizures
- May help to improve the efficacy of cancer treatment
- Improves cognitive function and memory recovery, particularly in Alzheimer's patients
- May reduce risk for heart disease and improve blood pressure
- Can help to reduce or treat severe breakouts and other skin conditions

Note: While you may be familiar with low-carbohydrate diets, the ketogenic diet is different in that it is not a fad diet – this type of diet is designed to provide your body with very real health benefits. If you are curious about trying the ketogenic diet for yourself you will find valuable information about what foods to include and avoid in your diet in the next chapter.

Chapter Two: The Ketogenic Diet

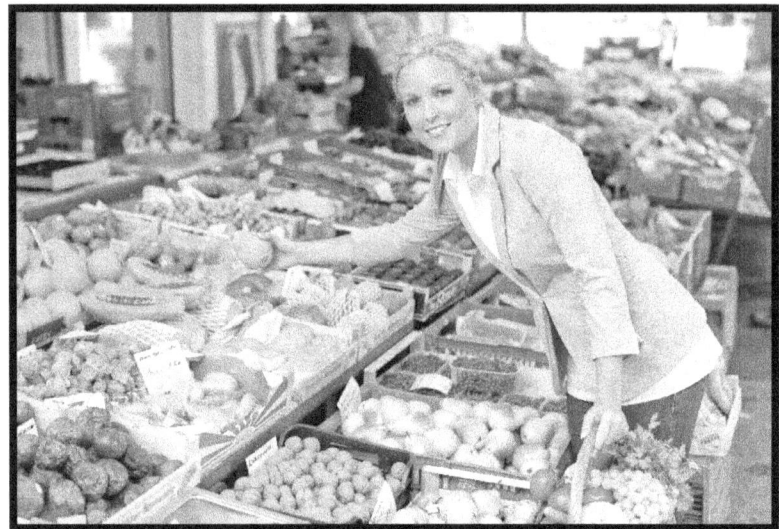

The ketogenic diet is more than just another fad diet designed to trick you into thinking that you might lose weight quickly by following some magical formula. In reality, the ketogenic diet was originally designed to treat a number of medical conditions including epilepsy, Type 2 diabetes and cancer. Numerous studies have indicated the beneficial effects of eating a low-carbohydrate, high-fat diet with adequate protein (see the benefits listed in the previous chapter). But how exactly does a ketogenic diet provide these benefits? When you consume carbohydrates, your body breaks down the food into its most basic components – glucose particles. The glucose is then transported throughout the body as fuel for vital processes. Excess glucose is stored in the cells and tissue as fat (glycogen) which can lead to a number of medical problems.

In following a low-carbohydrate (ketogenic) diet, the amount of stored glycogen in your body will decrease. As a result, your liver will begin to produce ketone bodies from the fats that you consume. These ketone bodies act as a replacement energy source and, when they pass into the brain, they can have a therapeutic effect on the body. A classic ketogenic diet involves consuming a 4:1 ratio of fat to combined protein and carbohydrate. In order to achieve this ratio, you must avoid high-carbohydrate foods and increase your consumption of high-fat foods. Though there are many variations of the ketogenic diet, it is generally recommended that you only consume foods that have a glycemic index below 50 and that you consume no more than 50 to 60 grams of carbohydrate per day.

Creating a Ketogenic Diet

In order to truly follow the ketogenic diet, you must do more than simply reduce your intake of carbohydrates – you have to think about what foods you are eating and why you are eating them. The glycemic index is a rating system assigned to carbohydrate-rich foods based on the effect they have on blood glucose levels after consumption. Foods with a high glycemic index (GI) rating have a higher impact on blood glucose levels while foods with a low GI rating have a lower impact. For example, starchy foods like bread and pasta are high-GI foods while vegetables, nuts and seeds are low-GI foods. To follow the ketogenic diet, you should avoid foods that contain a glycemic index above 50.

Some of the most popular foods having a GI rating above 50 include:

• Enriched grains	• Soft drinks	• Potato chips
• Pita bread	• Beer	• Candy
• Basmati rice	• Commercial cereals	• Ice cream
• White rice	• Pasta	• Table sugar
• Potatoes	• Pastries	
• White bread	• Cookies and cake	

Foods with a Low GI Rating (55 or less) include:

These are foods that you can enjoy in moderation while following the ketogenic diet, provided you consume no more than 50 to 60 grams of carbs daily.

• White beans	• Black Beans	• Kidney beans

- Navy beans
- Lentils
- Chickpeas
- Peanuts
- Almonds
- Walnuts
- Cashews
- Sunflower seeds
- Flaxseed
- Pumpkin seeds
- Sesame seeds
- Whole grains
- Rolled oats
- Barley
- Almond milk
- Greek yogurt

- Dairy milk
- Soy milk
- Peaches
- Mango
- Plums
- Blackberries
- Raspberries
- Strawberries
- Oranges
- Nectarines
- Apricot
- Grapefruit
- Pears
- Banana
- Mushrooms
- Artichoke

- Asparagus
- Bean sprouts
- Broccoli
- Cauliflower
- Cabbage
- Celery
- Cucumber
- Eggplant
- Lettuce
- Leafy greens
- Onions
- Radishes
- Squash
- Tomato
- Zucchini

Foods that Contain Primarily Fat, Protein and Water

These foods are no- or low-carbohydrate foods that should form the foundation of your ketogenic diet.

- Eggs
- Chicken
- Turkey
- Beef
- Pork
- Veal
- Game meat
- Fish
- Shrimp
- Scallops

- Mussels
- Clams
- Crab
- Lobster
- Tofu
- Olive oil
- Coconut oil
- Avocado
- Avocado oil
- Sesame seed oil

- Flaxseed oil
- Palm oil
- Mushrooms
- Artichoke
- Asparagus
- Bean sprouts
- Broccoli
- Cauliflower
- Cabbage
- Celery

- Cucumber
- Eggplant
- Lettuce

- Leafy greens
- Onions
- Radishes

- Squash
- Tomato
- Zucchini

Note: While the ketogenic diet is a high-fat diet, that doesn't mean you should be eating unhealthy fats. Your diet should be centered on heart-healthy monosaturated fats that come from natural sources like avocado, olives and olive oil. Avoid processed vegetable oils and hydrogenated oils as well as other forms of trans-fats.

Chapter Three: Ketogenic Recipes

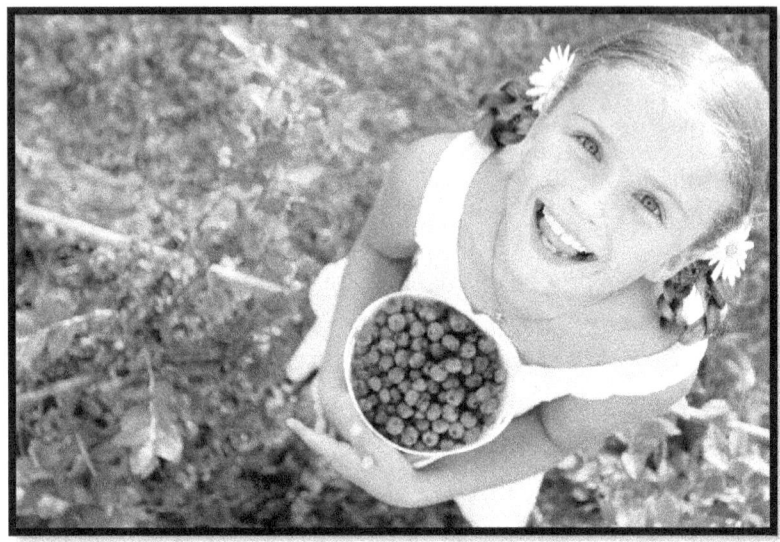

Recipes Included in this Book:

Spiced Pumpkin Waffles

Herbed Mushroom Omelet

Almond Flour Blueberry Muffins

Garlic Cheddar Biscuits

Walnut, Apple Chicken Salad

Creamy Avocado Soup

Avocado Egg Salad

Curried Lentil Soup

Herb-Roasted Chicken Legs

Balsamic Grilled Salmon Steaks

Cheese-Stuffed Meatloaf

Bacon-Wrapped Scallops

Spiced Pumpkin Waffles

Servings: 6

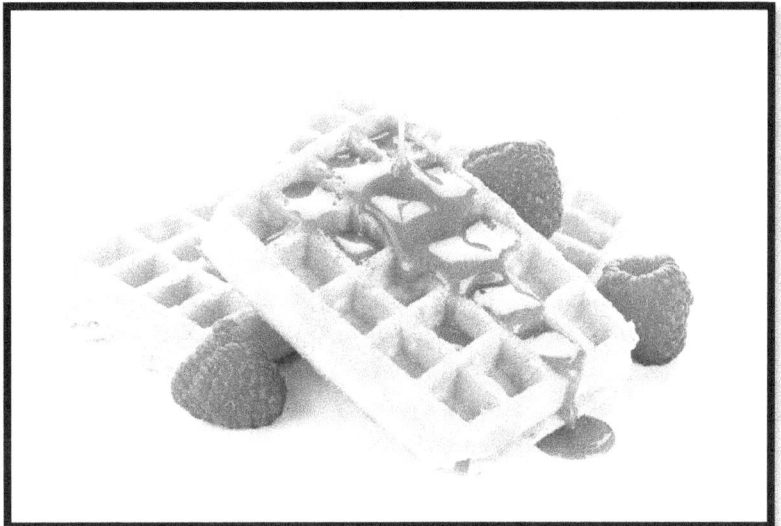

Ingredients:

- 1 cup pumpkin puree
- 6 large eggs, lightly whisked
- ½ cup unsweetened coconut milk
- ¼ cup coconut oil
- ¼ cup raw honey
- 1 ¾ cups almond flour
- 1/3 cup coconut flour
- 1 ½ teaspoons baking soda
- 1 teaspoon ground cinnamon

Instructions:

1. Grease and preheat your waffle iron.
2. Combine the pumpkin, eggs, coconut milk, coconut oil, honey and almond extract in a mixing bowl.
3. Whisk until smooth and well combined.

4. In a separate bowl, whisk together the almond flour, coconut flour, baking soda and cinnamon.

5. Add the dry ingredients to the wet and whisk until smooth.

6. Spoon about ¼ cup of batter into the waffle iron and cook according to the manufacturer's instructions.

Herbed Mushroom Omelet

Servings: 1

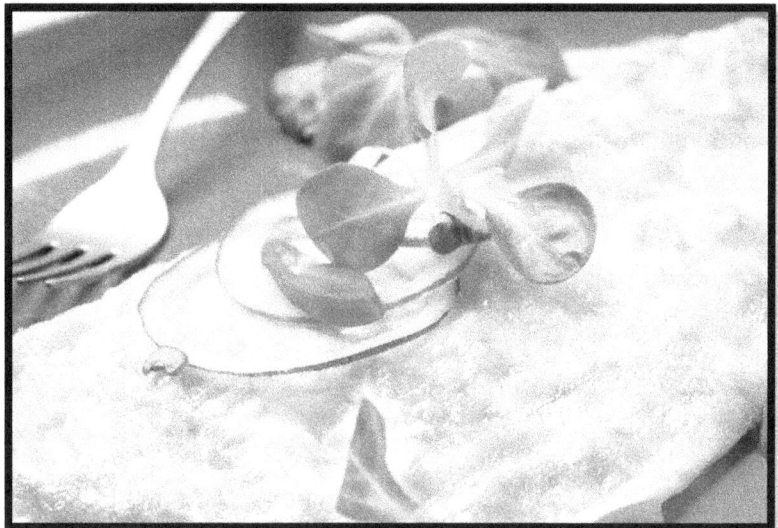

Ingredients:

- 2 teaspoons olive oil, divided
- 1 cup diced mushrooms
- 2 teaspoons fresh chopped basil
- 2 teaspoons fresh chopped parsley
- ¼ teaspoon dried oregano
- Salt and pepper to taste
- 2 large eggs
- 1 tablespoon skim milk
- 1 tablespoon fresh chopped chives

Instructions:

1. Heat 1 teaspoon olive oil in a small skillet over medium heat.
2. Add the mushrooms, basil, parsley and oregano. Season with salt and pepper to taste.
3. Cook for 2 to 3 minutes until the mushrooms are tender then spoon into a bowl.
4. Reheat the skillet with the remaining olive oil.

5. Whisk together the eggs, milk and chives in a small bowl then pour into the skillet.

6. Let cook for 1 minute then scrape down the sides of the skillet to spread the uncooked egg.

7. Cook for another 1 to 2 minutes until the egg is almost set.

8. Spoon the mushroom herb mixture over half the omelet and fold the empty half of the omelet over top.

9. Cook for 1 minute until the egg is set then slide onto a plate to serve.

Almond Flour Blueberry Muffins

Servings: 12

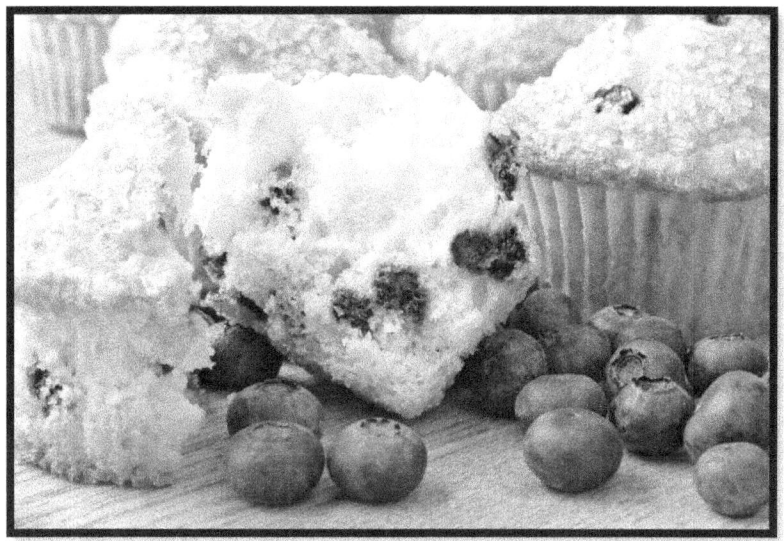

Ingredients:

- 1 ¼ cups almond flour
- 1 cup plus 1 tablespoon sorghum flour
- ½ cup tapioca starch
- ½ teaspoon salt
- 1 teaspoon baking powder
- ½ teaspoon baking soda
- 1 teaspoon xanthan gum
- 1 ¼ cups light brown sugar, packed
- 2 tablespoons olive oil
- 2 large eggs, lightly whisked
- ½ cup warm water
- 2 teaspoons vanilla extract

Instructions:

1. Preheat the oven to 375°F and line a muffin tin with paper liners.

2. Combine the flours, salt, baking soda, baking powder and xanthan gum in a large mixing bowl.

3. In a separate bowl, beat together the sugar, olive oil, eggs, water, and vanilla extract.

4. Add the dry ingredients to the wet in small batches and whisk until smooth.

5. Fold in the blueberries then spoon the batter into the prepared pan, filling each cup about ¾ full.

6. Bake for 22 to 25 minutes until lightly browned.

7. Cool in the pan for 5 minutes then turn out onto a wire rack to cool completely.

Garlic Cheddar Biscuits

Servings: 16

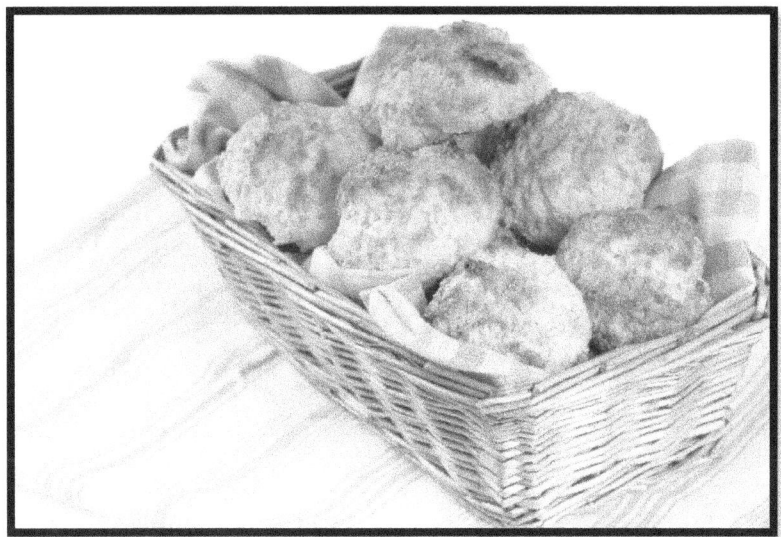

Ingredients:

- 1 ½ cups almond flour, divided
- 3 ounces shredded cheddar cheese
- 2 ½ tablespoons unsalted butter, softened
- 4 ounces cream cheese, softened
- 2 large egg, lightly whisked
- 1 teaspoon garlic powder
- ½ teaspoon baking soda
- ¼ teaspoon xanthan gum
- Pinch salt

Instructions:

1. Preheat the oven to 325°F and line a baking sheet with parchment paper.
2. Combine ½ cup almond flour with the shredded cheese and pulse until finely blended.
3. In a mixing bowl, beat together the butter and cream cheese.

4. Add the eggs, garlic, baking soda, xanthan gum and salt then whisk until smooth and well combined.

5. Whisk in the almond flour/cheddar cheese mixture and stir until it forms a sticky dough.

6. Drop the dough in heaping tablespoons onto the prepared baking sheet, spacing them about 1 inch apart.

7. Bake for 20 to 25 minutes until lightly browned. Cool for 10 minutes before serving.

Walnut, Apple Chicken Salad

Servings: 4

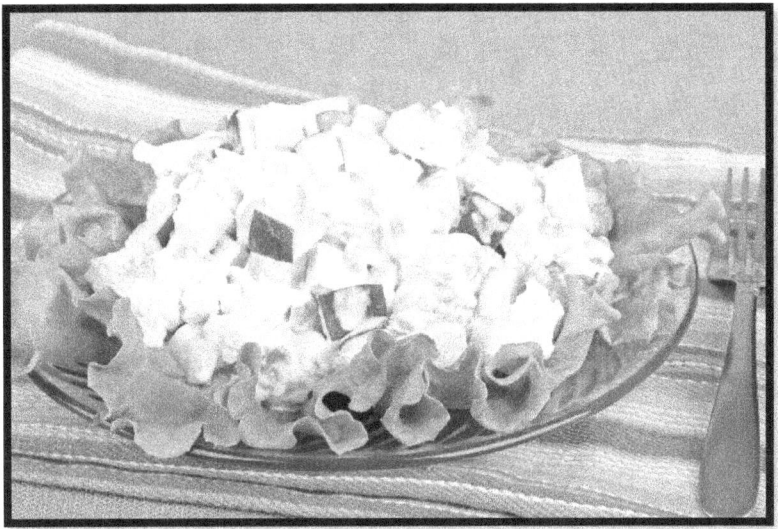

Ingredients:

- 2 boneless skinless chicken breasts, cooked and chopped
- 1 medium apple, finely chopped
- ¼ cup chopped walnuts
- ¼ cup diced celery
- ¼ cup olive oil
- 2 tablespoons fresh lemon juice
- 2 tablespoons minced red onion
- Salt and pepper to taste

Instructions:

1. Combine the chicken, apples, walnuts and celery in a mixing bowl.
2. Add the remaining ingredients and toss well to coat.
3. Cover and chill until ready to serve.

Creamy Avocado Soup

Servings: 6

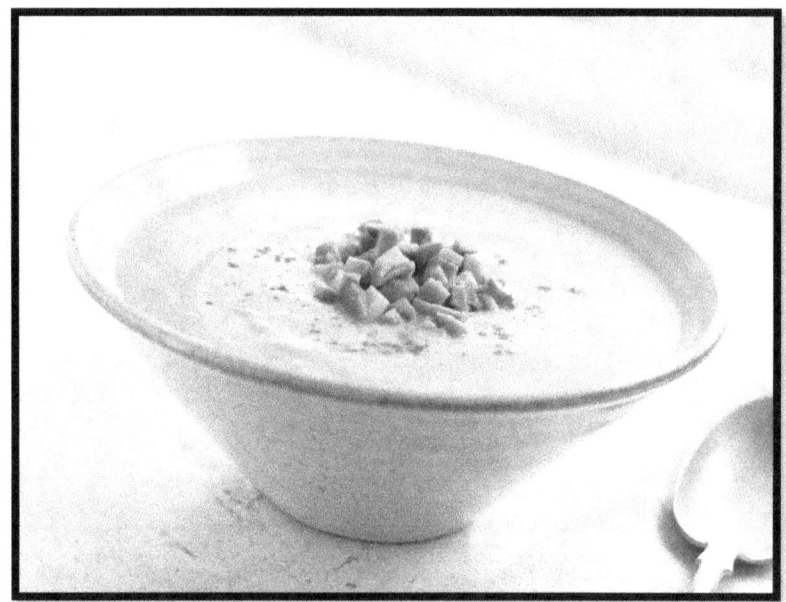

Ingredients:

- 4 ripe avocados, pitted and chopped
- 2 (14.5-ounce) cans chicken broth
- 2/3 cup canned coconut milk
- 2 shallots, finely diced
- 2 tablespoons dry white wine
- Pinch salt

Instructions:

1. Combine all of the ingredients in a food processor or blender.
2. Blend until smooth and well combined.
3. Pour the soup into a bowl then cover and chill for at least 6 hours before serving.
4. Garnish with diced avocado and a sprinkle of paprika to serve.

Avocado Egg Salad

Servings: 6

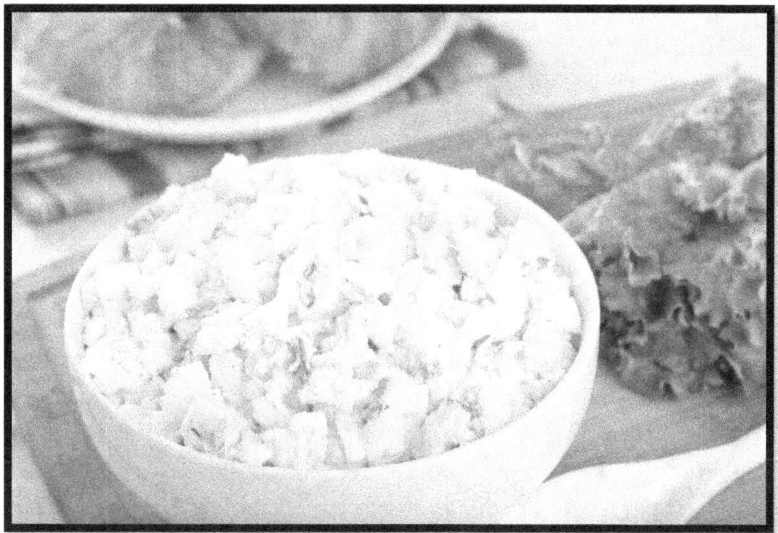

Ingredients:

- 4 large hardboiled eggs, whites and yolks divided
- 1 medium ripe avocado, pitted and diced
- 1 tablespoon mayonnaise
- 1 tablespoon non-fat yogurt, plain
- 2 teaspoons white wine vinegar
- 1 tablespoon fresh chopped chives
- Salt and pepper to taste

Instructions:

1. Chop the egg whites and set them aside.
2. Combine the egg yolks, avocado, mayonnaise, yogurt, vinegar and chives in a mixing bowl.
3. Mash the mixture well with a fork.
4. Season with salt and pepper to taste then fold in the chopped egg whites.
5. Adjust seasoning to taste and chill until ready to serve.

Curried Lentil Soup

Servings: 6

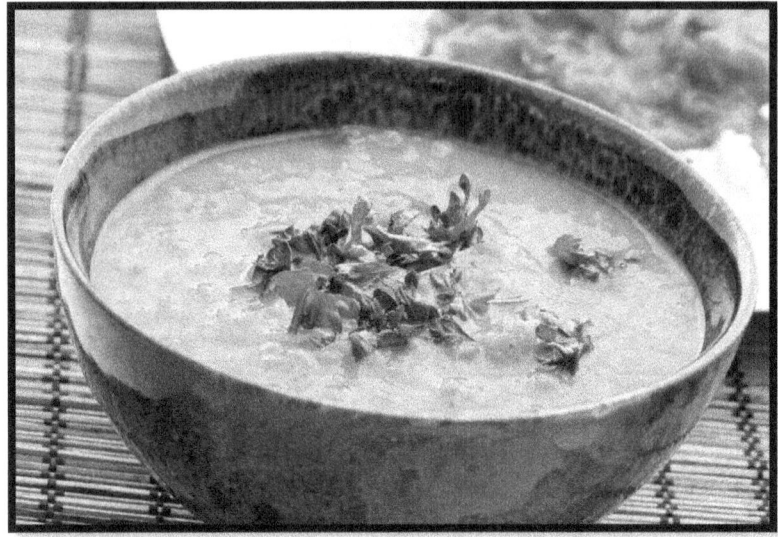

Ingredients:

- 1 tablespoon coconut oil
- 1 cup chopped onion
- ½ cup chopped carrot
- 1 teaspoon minced garlic
- Salt and pepper to taste
- 2 tablespoons curry powder
- 1 cup dry red lentils
- 4 cups water
- 1 (15-ounce) can chickpeas, rinsed and drained
- 1 tablespoon fresh lemon juice
- 2 tablespoons olive oil

Instructions:

1. Heat the coconut oil in a large stockpot over medium heat.
2. Add the carrot and onion then stir in the salt and pepper to taste.

3. Cook for 4 to 6 minutes until the onions are translucent then stir in the garlic.

4. Let the mixture cook for another 3 minutes or so.

5. Stir in the curry powder, lentils and water.

6. Bring to a boil then reduce heat and simmer for 30 minutes until the lentils are tender.

7. Combine the chickpeas, lemon juice and olive oil in a food processor then stir into the stockpot.

8. Let the soup cook until heated through then adjust seasonings to taste before serving hot.

Herb-Roasted Chicken Legs

Servings: 6

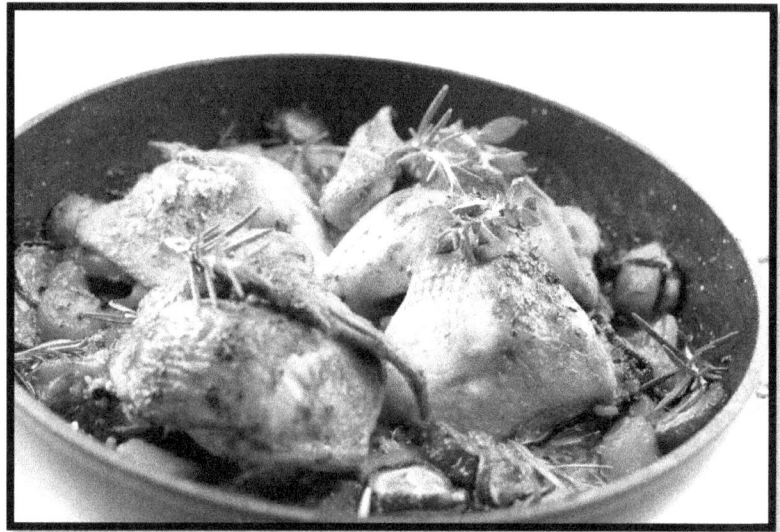

Ingredients:

- 2 lbs. bone-in chicken legs
- 2 tablespoons coconut oil
- Salt and pepper to taste
- 2 large onions, coarsely chopped
- 1 tablespoon dried rosemary
- 1 teaspoon dried oregano
- ½ teaspoon dried thyme
- ¼ cup chicken broth

Instructions:

1. Preheat the oven to 400°F.
2. Liberally season the chicken legs with salt and pepper on both sides.
3. Heat the oil in a large skillet and add the chicken – cook for 2 to 3 minutes on each side until evenly browned.
4. Spread the onions in a large glass baking dish and place the chicken on top.

5. Combine the rosemary, oregano and thyme in a small bowl then sprinkle over the chicken and onions.

6. Drizzle with broth then roast for 30 minutes.

7. Carefully turn the chicken then roast for another 25 to 30 minutes until the juices run clear. Serve hot.

Balsamic Grilled Salmon Steaks

Servings: 4

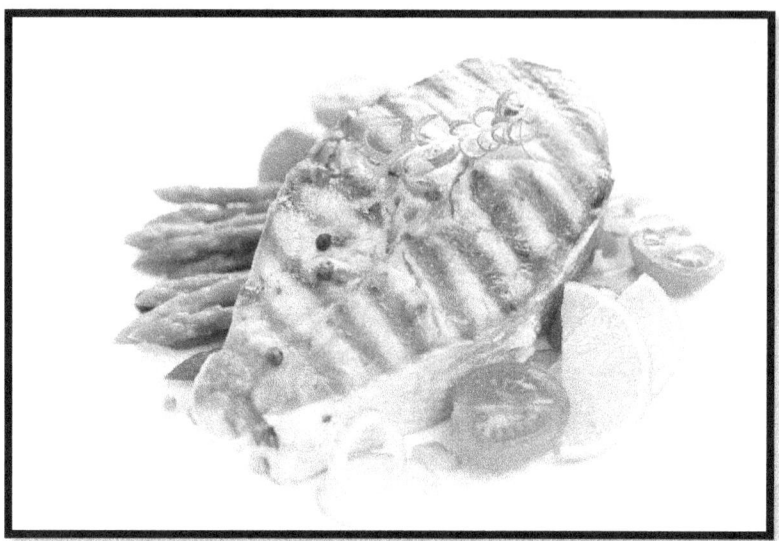

Ingredients:

- 4 (6-ounce) boneless salmon steaks
- 2 tablespoons olive oil
- 1 tablespoon white wine vinegar
- 1 tablespoon balsamic vinegar
- 1 teaspoon sugar
- Salt and pepper to taste

Instructions:

1. Whisk together the oil, vinegars, sugar, salt and pepper in a small bowl.
2. Place the salmon in a large re-sealable freezer bag and pour in the marinade.
3. Toss to coat then chill for 1 hour, turning occasionally.
4. Preheat your grill to high heat then turn the heat down to medium.
5. Add the salmon steaks and grill for 4 to 6 minutes on each side until seared. Serve hot.

Cheese-Stuffed Meatloaf

Servings: 10 to 12

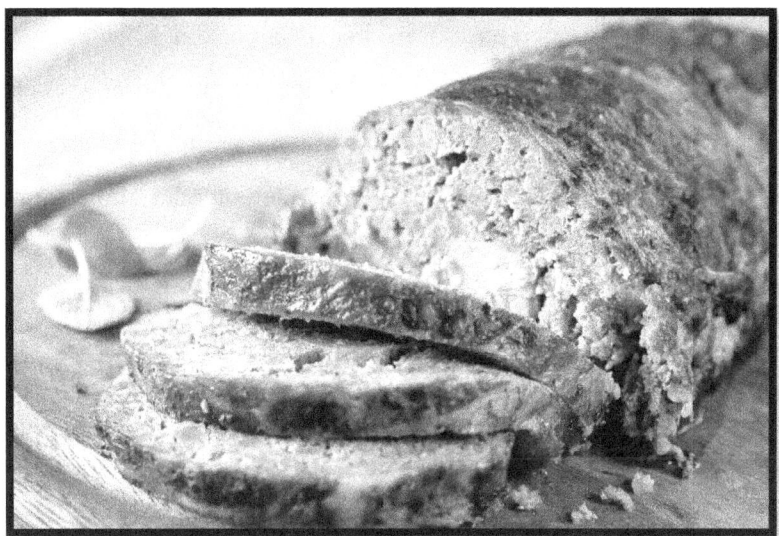

Ingredients:

- 1 (8-ounce) package cream cheese, softened
- 2 cups shredded cheddar cheese
- ½ cup almond flour
- ½ cup grated parmesan cheese
- 1 cup chopped yellow onion
- 1 tablespoon minced garlic
- 1 teaspoon salt
- ½ teaspoon pepper
- 2 large eggs, lightly whisked
- 2 tablespoons ketchup
- ¼ cup heavy cream
- 2 lbs. lean ground beef
- 1 lbs. ground pork

Instructions:

1. Preheat the oven to 350°F and lightly grease a glass baking dish.

2. Combine the cream cheese and shredded cheddar cheese in a mixing bowl and stir until soft and smooth. Set aside.

3. Stir together the almond flour and parmesan cheese. Set aside.

4. Place the onion, garlic, salt and pepper in a food processor and blend until pureed.

5. In a deep bowl, whisk together the eggs with the onion mixture, ketchup and cream. Stir well.

6. Combine the ground beef and pork in a mixing bowl then blend in the egg mixture by hand.

7. Add the almond flour mixture and blend well.

8. Transfer the meat mixture to a parchment-lined baking sheet and spread into an even slap.

9. Spread the cream cheese mixture over the meat then use the parchment paper to roll the meat into a log.

10. Transfer the loaf to the greased baking dish and bake for 1 hour or until the internal temperature reaches 160°F.

11. Let the meatloaf rest for 10 minutes before slicing.

Bacon-Wrapped Scallops

Servings: 4

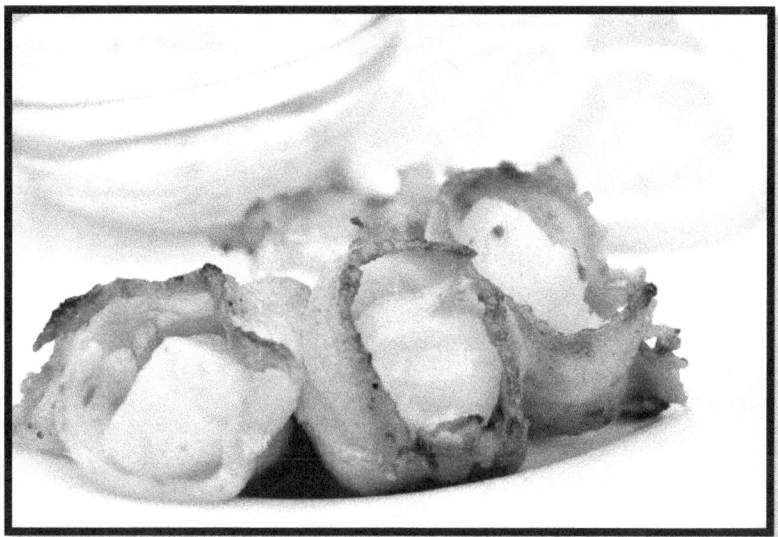

Ingredients:

- 1 ¼ lbs. raw sea scallops
- ½ to ¾ lbs. uncooked bacon
- 1 teaspoon chili powder
- ½ teaspoon black pepper
- ¼ teaspoon salt
- ¼ teaspoon paprika

Instructions:

1. Preheat the broiler in your oven to high heat.
2. Rinse the scallops in cool water then pat dry and arrange on a broiler pan.
3. Combine the chili powder, pepper, salt and paprika in a small bowl then sprinkle over the scallops.
4. Wrap each scallop in a slice of bacon and secure in place with a wooden toothpick.
5. Broil the scallops for 4 to 5 minutes on each side until the bacon is crisp and cooked through.

Conclusion

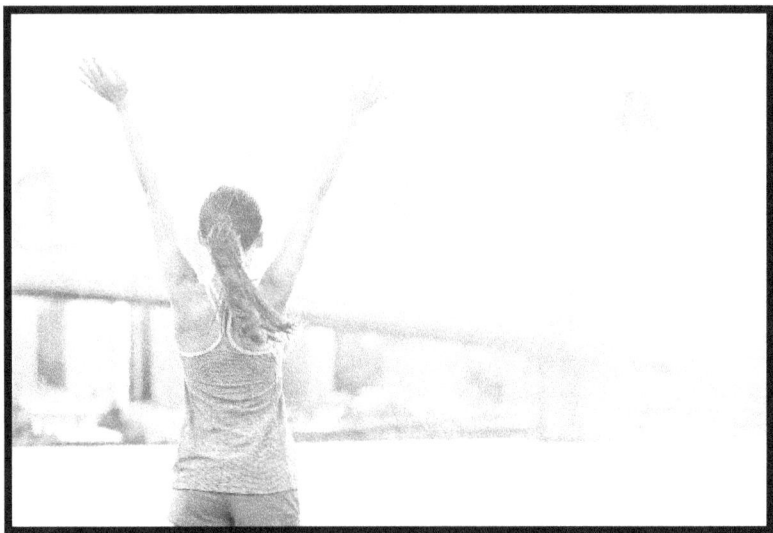

After reading this book you should have a good idea what ketosis is and how it can benefit your body. You have also learned the basics about the ketogenic diet and what type of foods you should eat on this diet, as well as what foods to avoid. In addition to this basic information, you also received a collection of ketogenic diet recipes to get you started on your new diet. Hopefully this book has provided you with the information you need to understand and get started on your new diet so you can be on your way to achieving a happier, healthier you.

Thanks for reading and good luck with your ketogenic diet!

www.ingramcontent.com/pod-product-compliance
Lightning Source LLC
Chambersburg PA
CBHW081809280526
45789CB00008B/3065